The Allergy Saving Book

A Complete Guide to Solving Food Sensitivities and
Related Health Problems

By: Martha Grace Hart

9781681275147

PUBLISHERS NOTES

Disclaimer – Speedy Publishing LLC

This publication is intended to provide helpful and informative material. It is not intended to diagnose, treat, cure, or prevent any health problem or condition, nor is intended to replace the advice of a physician. No action should be taken solely on the contents of this book. Always consult your physician or qualified health-care professional on any matters regarding your health and before adopting any suggestions in this book or drawing inferences from it.

The author and publisher specifically disclaim all responsibility for any liability, loss or risk, personal or otherwise, which is incurred as a consequence, directly or indirectly, from the use or application of any contents of this book.

Any and all product names referenced within this book are the trademarks of their respective owners. None of these owners have sponsored, authorized, endorsed, or approved this book.

Always read all information provided by the manufacturers' product labels before using their products. The author and publisher are not responsible for claims made by manufacturers.

This book was originally printed before 2014. This is an adapted reprint by Speedy Publishing LLC with newly updated content designed to help readers with much more accurate and timely information and data.

Speedy Publishing LLC

40 E Main Street, Newark, Delaware, 19711

Contact Us: 1-888-248-4521

Website: http://www.speedypublishing.co

REPRINTED Paperback Edition: 9781681275147:

Manufactured in the United States of America

DEDICATION

This book is dedicated to Gerard. You have no idea how much you mean to me. Because of you, I became a nurse, a teacher, a friend, a playmate and most of all, a mother.

TABLE OF CONTENTS

CHAPTER 1- WHAT CAUSES ALLERGIES?

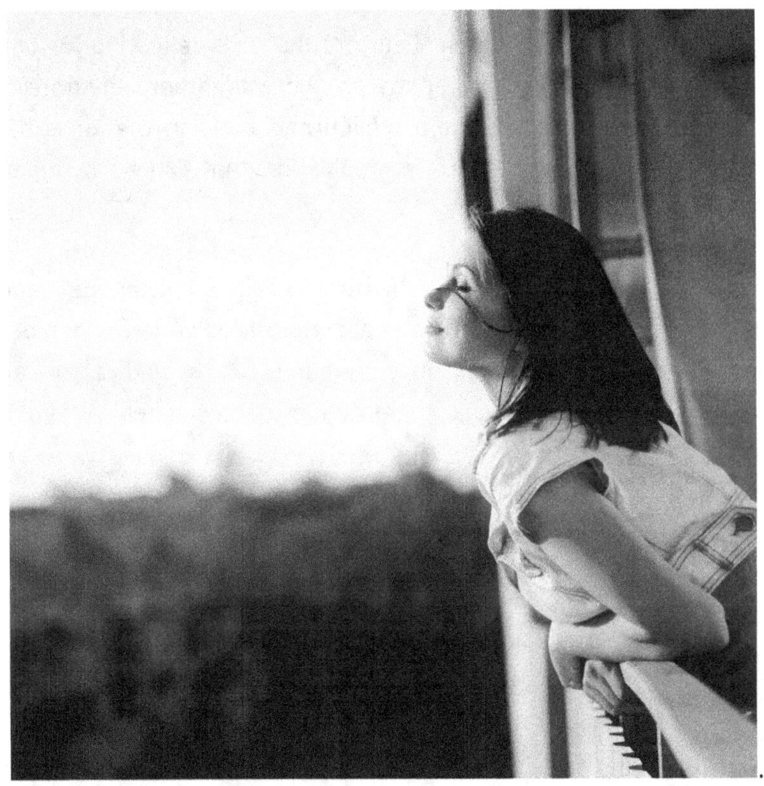

Allergies are annoying creatures that sneak up on us when the weather changes. In our home we fight allergies, since mold, germs, pollen, dust, dust mites and so on hide in cracks and corners. We don't realize it but each night we lie down in our bed, we have dust mites hiding beneath the covers.

More than 5,000 people in the US alone suffer from allergies, including hay fever, asthma sinus infections and so on. Most of these people suffer aggravating conditions that interrupt their lifestyle. Most seek medical help from doctors, yet in most instances they continue to suffer despite their efforts to slow allergies.

People have allergy problems year around. It is called indoor and outdoor allergies. Nasal allergies are very common anymore it seems like everyone has them. Pollen and mold in the air is the cause for allergies and there is medication that can be taken to help but not cure allergies.

Our body produces two chemicals called histamine and leukotrienes and these are both allergies. Medication can block these so your body can't produce so many. Taking medication can give you fun time for a picnic, be more alert, and can help you get a better night of sleep.

Symptoms for allergies include:

• Runny eyes

• Sneezing

• Coughing

• Stuffy nose

• Rash

• Breathing Problems

You might want to check with your doctor before starting any treatment on your own. He might have a different treatment he'll want to try before using an over the counter drug.

There are many different medications, which can be taken to help you enjoy your life without having to feel down because of allergies. Some medicine comes in a spray to spray into your nose and there are some just for stuffiness. Be sure to read all labels to make sure you aren't allergic to any of the ingredients and make notice if it is non-drowsy or not. Allergy medications work on blocking the histamine from producing more and faster. Ask your family physician about trying a medication that is taken year around to prevent your allergies from popping up on you.

Knowing the pollen pattern and when it is going to hit your area is one way to start treatment before the allergies hit you. You can get on the Internet and search for allergies to find the site for you. They will send you e-mail and let you know 4 weeks before the allergy season is going to hit your town.

Keeping an ongoing list of allergies or what triggers them will help you a lot. If you know what allergies, you have than you can try to avoid them. By avoiding things you know will trigger you allergies you'll feel better.

Some people often have to see a specialist who can detect what allergies they might have. Talk to your family physician and see how he feels if your treatments that your currently doing doesn't seem to be helping.

By knowing exactly what allergies you have it will be a lot easier to avoid being around them and they can be treated easier.

If you have upholstered furniture and carpets, try removing as much as possible. Carpets and upholstered furniture collect dust and pollens that float in the air. You can buy a special spray for the ones that you aren't able to get rid of. Cleaning for your carpets and furniture is very important to keep the dust out of them.

Check your mattress on the beds and spray them too. Get you a mattress cover with a zipper in it to keep the dust off. It is a lot easier to take a damp cloth and dust over the mattress every couple of days that spraying all around it and cheaper too.

Using air-filtering techniques to help reduce the dust and pollen that is floating through the air in your home can help reduce allergic-based pollutions. Do some research on the Internet and check out the best that fits your needs. Air filters come in all different brand names, sizes, styles and prices to make things easier on you and your wallet.

Pets are another one for carrying dust mites. Keep them out of the bedrooms and off the furniture. Some people have been known to have to get rid of their pets because of their allergies.

Many ways are available to cut down the dust and pollen that goes along with allergies so research is a good way to help reduce allergies to be healthier. Learn more about environment and how it affects you also.

Dust Mites and Allergies

Dust mites can hide. They are not seen by the human eye. To avoid these critters you will need to consider bedding and furniture that is not made up upholstery types of material. Foam is recommended. However, you can purchase bedding, such as pillowcases, blankets, and sheets and so on to reduce dust mites.

Dust mites cannot survive in climates below 39 degrees. We certainly do not want a home with this level of coolness. Still, we can use dehumidifiers, purifiers and humidifiers to keep dust mites at bay.

Dust mites can cause swelling eyes, running nose, congestion, headaches and so on. The allergic symptoms emerging from dust mites affects over 80% of those diagnosed with allergies and most do not know that they are allergic to these spider mites.

To learn more about these mites visit your doctor. Your doctor will provide you with pamphlets or other information related to these allergic conditions. Most doctors today are studying allergies stronger than at one time, since allergic problems is hitting the charts and causing serious illnesses to emerge.

The Importance of a Healthy Home Environment

Home environment is very important to be concerned with for allergy treatment. Reducing the animal dander, dust mites, mold and pollen will help with the allergy problems and help to keep you healthy. Keeping the home clean is one of the key words for allergy relief.

Getting rid of the allergens or neutralize them is very important. When neutral these harmful items from the house it is harmless when it is inhaled. Treating the carpets, furniture, and bedding regularly is the best way to neutralize the allergens in your home.

Neutralizing your home can be done with many different products. They come in sprays, powder and then vacuum, carpet cleaners and even laundry detergent. These items can be bought at hardware stores, health stores and on the Internet too. Do some research on the Internet where you'll find articles on different items to use when neutralizing your home?

Mold and mildew are a major problem for people with allergies and it can be very harmful to your immune system. Avoid having mold and mildew to keep yourself and those around you in good health.

There are special products out to get rid of just mold and mildew and they come in many different powders and sprays. Check out the products and get the one that will do the job for you and your family's health.

The pets and odors in your home need to be kept clean and free of allergen free. Make use when buying your pet supplies that it is the right one to rid your home of dust mites and animal allergen. There are so many kinds of pet supplies out now for the pet in your home to help keep your family in the allergen free home environment.

When buying your laundry supplies to keep the allergens down in the home, be sure to read the labels. You need one for people that are sensitive to allergies. Your laundry detergent should be free from perfume, bleach and any harsh chemicals. These can even be used in hot or cold water.

Controlling the mold and dust mites can partly be done with humidity control in the home. Dust mites with die when the humidity is below 50%. Mold lives for humidity so keeping it low with kill the mold if it is high it spreads more. The dust mites will stay alive in your bedding by living off the sheds of skin from your body so be sure to keep the mattress, box springs, and pillows encased with a zipper closing.

Vacuuming the carpet and furniture should be done two or 3 times a week to help reduce the allergens in the home.

A vacuum sweeper with a filter is most recommended for the great amount of allergens it takes out of the air. Instead of seeing dust fly from your sweeper as you commonly do with ordinary vacuums, check out the filtered sweepers. The filtered vacuums are sold most anywhere that vacuum sweepers are sold with many different brands, styles and prices. Your vacuum should include attachments for cleaning those hard to get space in the corners and to do your furniture with. Dust mites are everywhere so, be sure to get under you cushions too.

Air filtrations are something every home needs to keep the air clean of all those dust mites flying around. Breathing fresh air is important for especially people with allergies. When going to buy one be sure to know your room size and get one based for that room or larger. The larger your unit is the better cleaning job it will do for you.

Keep your home environment clean and everyone will be healthier.

Keeping the Home Air Clean

With the outside air being more polluted all the time, more people are getting allergies every day. When the air outside is polluted, it is 100 times worse inside. Most people spend more time inside where the air is worse than outside in fresh air.

Home environment is very important for people with allergies and the health of all your loved ones too. Get some cleaning done with an air filter today.

Poor air is not good for healthy people. It causes them to have headaches, fatigue, and irritation to the eyes, nose and throat. Your loved ones with allergy and respiratory problems need clean air to help them live a more normal life.

Air filters are used inside your home to clean out the air pollution that is floating around. Using air filters will turn your air to crisp and clean air along with removing the bacteria, mole, virus and fungi. Your home will smell better and you will have less dusting to do.

Eliminating harmful odors such as paint smell, aerosol sprays and cleaning supplies are important and using a good air filter in the home can do this. Air filters break down the chemicals by breaking down the pollution eliminating many serious health issues.

There are many different kinds of air filters and sizes. You need to shop around to find the one to best fit the needs and air around you. Choosing an air filter is choosing the best one to fit best.

You might want to consider getting a small air filter for the bedrooms first. When you are sleeping, is when you need the cleanest air. The human respiratory system slows down when you are sleeping and can't handle the pollution as well as it can during the day. With a filter in your bedroom you will have a longer period to breathe in clean air, letting you wake up in the morning feeling more refreshed and less congested.

Air purifiers need to be running 24 hours a day to do what is expected from them. If you don't have enough money to buy, only for the bedrooms it is very important that you moved it out to the living area during the day to clean that air. Air floats and the pollution will go from one room to another so keeping the air clean at all times is important.

Thinking about why you are buying an air filter will help you decide on the best one to fit your needs. People buy them just to keep the air clean for the new baby room, to clean the mold from returning, for the pet odors or specific health reasons.

Once you know why you're buying an air purifier for your home then buying the best one will come easy. Air purifiers come in many different styles so choose one for the specific reason you are buying.

Buying air purifiers are not always the solution for people with allergies. As winter leaves, we're glad to see warmer weather but dreading the allergies that come with spring.

Contacting your doctor is the first thing you need to do and get prepared. Ask your doctor for all the new information he can give you for allergies, contact your health insurance and see if they have a health calendar with dates that the pollution is in its high peek of the season.

You can go on the Internet and go to the weather site to find out where and when the high pollution season is and in what area when planning a vacation. Have your medications close at hand; the long term ones and the quick fixes if needed, and have the calendar where you can look ahead to see what is headed to your area during the high pollution seasons. Preparing for allergy season is just as important as buying an air purifier. Elimination for allergy relief is possible when you take action.

CHAPTER 2- ASTHMA, COPD AND OTHER RESPIRATORY PROBLEMS

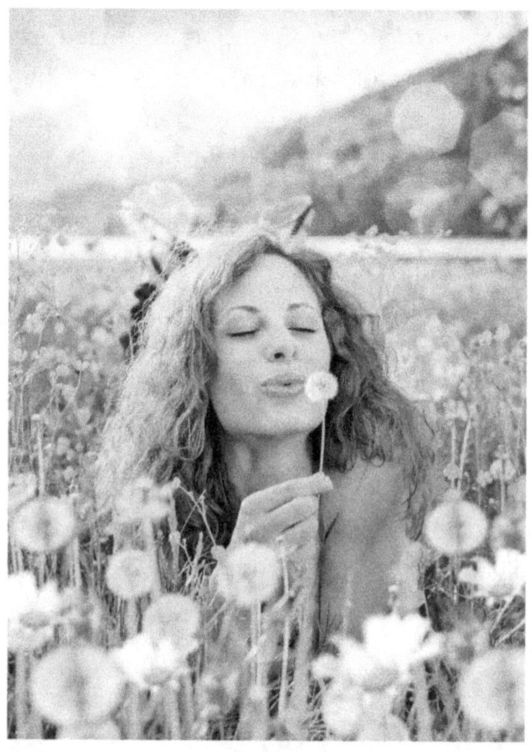

The respiratory system plays a large part in allergy relief. When you battle allergies, you will need to follow-up with your doctor appointments. Your doctor will need to monitor the condition and treatment to see where it goes.

To find allergy relief you will need to avoid irritants that cause allergy attacks. Smoking is one of the irritants you will need to stop to find relief of allergies, or asthma attacks.

Other irritants may include dust, pollen, mildew, mold, pet dander, dust mites and so on. You will need to learn cleaning tips to keep these irritants at bay. Dust mites are controlled with humidifiers, dehumidifiers, air conditioners, plastic, and so on. Place plastic over your mattress and wash your sheets and blankets weekly to keep dust mites at bay. Dust each day and purchase products that help you control dust and other irritants in your home.

How doctor follow-up helps you:

When you follow-up with your doctor you will be instructed to self-monitor your symptoms. If you notice infections, you will need to visit your doctor to find relief. You will need to avoid people who may have infections to fight allergies.

How to control infections:

Once you notice distress of the respiratory and infections you will need to seek medical support. Your doctor may prescribe you an antibiotic to control the infection and upper respiratory condition.

How controlling weight helps you:

You can find allergy relief also by controlling your weight. If you have access weight exercise is a good way to keep the weight down.

How medications work for you:

Your doctor will need to prescribe medication to control severe allergy conditions, or asthma. The doctor will take action and work to avoid adverse medicine effects while setting up a schedule for medicine intake.

What makes some fruits and vegetables are hazardous?

You will need to set restrictions in dieting. Your doctor can help you learn what foods to avoid. If you are allergic to latex, you may want to avoid bananas, cherries, apricots, chestnuts, kiwi, nectarines, celery, pineapple, potatoes, plums, melons, avocados, rubber gloves, tomatoes, peaches, and grapes. These fruits and vegetables come from latex trees and vines. Rather, this material is where latex products come from, so avoiding these when allergic to latex will help you find allergy relief.

You will need to set up activities that help you control allergies and asthma also. Getting proper rest is a great way to control allergies. When you do not have proper rest, it can cause stress and allergies to emerge. If you have asthma, it will affect your health also.

How to find resources in allergy relief:

Resources are available to help you control allergies or to learn more about this condition.

When you have an understanding of your condition, it can help you find relief. You likely have community resources and agencies in your neighborhood. We encourage you to research your area to find out about these resources and agencies. The Internet offers you a wide assortment of free information as well. Go online and read some of the articles available to you. Technology has advanced, which means new medicines and allergy relief over-the-counter products are coming available. Learn more about these up-to-date products so that you can help your doctor find solutions that bring you allergy relief.

How asthma affects you:

Asthma can emerge from allergies. Allergies are a condition that stems from chronic obstructive pulmonary disease. (COPD)

If you have asthma, you want to follow-up with your doctor regularly, since asthma is life threatening. Don't take your life into your own hands when help is available.

More on Asthma

Studies show that children are affected by asthma, which the children miss millions of days at schools because of this condition. Each year billions of dollars are spent to care for allergy or asthma patients. Asthma has claimed more than 100,000 lives annually. Recently, experts found that asthma alone is far more dangerous than they once believed.

At one time experts believed that environmental irritants were responsible for asthma attacks. Yet, new studies were taken in areas where irritants declined and it showed that asthma continued to increase, taking lives, sending people to emergency rooms and so on.

Some of the evidence found in these studies pointed to medications prescribed to treat allergies and asthma. Since asthma and allergies, increased experts today are searching for answers in the latest allergy medications.

On this note, it seems we need yoga and other healthy activities into our daily living to avoid side effects from allergic-based drugs.

About COPD

Chronic obstructive pulmonary disease (COPD) causes asthma attacks, as well as allergy outbreaks. By definition, COPD is a cluster of disease that stem from unrelenting "obstruction of the bronchial air flow." The condition can cause you to suffer chronic bronchitis, bronchiectasis, asthma and emphysema. Smoking is the leading cause of these conditions, yet other irritants in our environment can cause the conditions to emerge also.

When you are battling disease, you will need to continue frequent follow-up with your doctor. Your doctor must know your symptoms. Tell your doctor when you visit everything you can about your condition. This will help the doctor find treatments that work for you. Your doctor will need to monitor you thereafter, so continue keeping your doctor appointments.

How emphysema affects you:

When a person is diagnosed with emphysema, it is one of the worst conditions related to allergies that you can endure. Emphysema causes a stimulation to affect your breathing pattern, which is a PO-2 commonly, i.e. low. PCO-2 decreases.

To find allergy relief you will need to avoid irritants, which in this case is smoke. You want to stay out of areas where people smoke, and avoid smoking tobacco.

What are the possibilities in etiology?

If you are diagnosed with asthma, emphysema or bronchial conditions your lungs can weaken. The respiratory system is irritated, which usually comes from chemical irritants, polluted air, or smoke. The condition leads to respiratory tract infections. Your doctor will need to monitor this condition often.

How can I determine what symptoms are related to these conditions?

If you have such conditions, you want to notice coughing, dyspnea, and usage of "accessory muscles," crackles, wheezing, exertional dyspnea and barrel chest. Sputum productions are observable when emphysema is present. Asthma or bronchial infections can present anxiousness, anemia, hemoptysis, weight loss, Orthopnea, diaphoresis, finger clubbing, malaise and so on.

If you have common allergies you want to avoid irritants in the environment, home, work and so on. Your condition could develop into chronic pulmonary systems in later years.

Some of the irritants to avoid include pollen, pet dander, dust mites, dust, and smoke, harsh chemicals, mold, mildew and so on. Other irritants that are made of latex can affect you also, especially if you are allergic to such products.

Bananas, cherries, apricots, nuts, chestnuts, kiwi, nectarines, celery, are all products that come from latex. Pineapple, plums, melons, potatoes, avocados, tomatoes, peaches, and grapes come from latex trees and shrubs also.

Fighting COPD and Allergies

If you are subject to such conditions speak with your doctor. Your doctor will help you avoid such conditions. You want to set a diet that provides you plenty Vitamin C, proteins, and if possible nitrogen. You will need to increase fluids daily to around "3,000 milligrams.

In addition, you want to keep your weight down. We all can benefit from exercise. Set up a schedule that works for you and exercise often. Exercise will help you maintain weight, and will reduce your risks of disease.

You will need a healthy diet. Learn more about what irritants your respiratory system so that you can stay away from these products.

Sometimes you have to move from your environment when allergies, asthma or other related conditions affect you. The environment may have irritants in the air that causes you distress. Talk to your doctor.

Some of us can benefit from a warm climate. Some people move to Arizona or other areas where pollutants in the air are less severe.

Chapter 3- Conquering Panic when Allergy Attacks

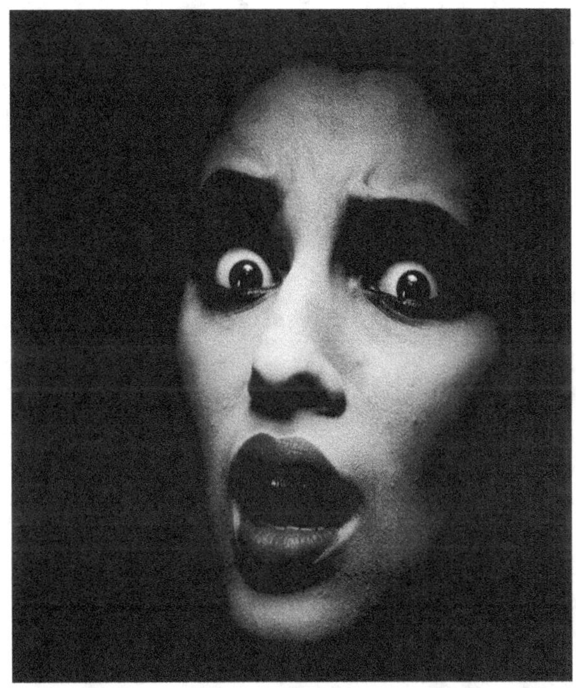

Breathing patterns are very important if you have allergies. When a person can't breathe, they begin to panic and learning how to control our breathing is necessary for everyone. Changing our breathing patterns can be done with little effort. Some practice and learning techniques will help us to take control of breathing.

Breathing comes natural from birth and as we age sometimes, it needs to be changed to keep us healthy. In order to change our pattern we need to understand a little bit how the breathing technique works.

How breathing, inhaling works:

As we inhale our brain, sends a message to the diaphragm that is the muscle separating the heart and lungs from the stomach. When the message gets to the diaphragm, it activates it. It will flatten out letting the lower ribs swing out so the chest cavity can increase. As the chest cavity, increases the lungs will pull air into the lower lungs.

How exhaling works:

When we exhale the lungs and muscles will go back to its normal size. After a pause, the process will start over again with the brain sending, it's message. The normal process of breathing is 14 times a minute more depending on how much the person needs it.

Breathing is controlled by the nervous system to run in its self-correcting mode. There are to branches of the self-correcting mode, one is "relaxation response" and the other is "fight response".

How the relaxation response works:

The relaxation response tells the system to slow the heart a breathing rate down. It works to keep the digestion and elimination going at the normal rate.

The fight response reacts to the functions that relate to emergencies and exercises. This response wakes and rouses our system to respond to the emergency by pumping adrenaline making our heart and breathing increases their rate. The increase will supply more oxygen to our bodies. If we are in real danger, the energy is used if not it could cause anxiety and hyperventilation.

How breathing fast affects you:

With allergies or asthma, we tend to breathe faster not realizing it. Breathing at a faster rate will take more energy out of us but letting us have more oxygen. At the same time, though when we breathe out we are losing too much carbon dioxide. If we lose too much carbon dioxide, it can be critical. The hemoglobin that carries the oxygen through our blood to the cells will become sticky not letting the oxygen through.

Learn to slow down your breathing rate to reduce your attacks. There are exercises that can be done to help you to breathe. Continue take all medications and consult your physician before starting to learn new breathing techniques.

Using Yoga to Relieve Allergy Symptoms

Studies showed that yoga could reduce allergies over 60%. Yoga helps keep away allergies, asthma, and hay fever and so on.

Allergies can cause you to wake during the night, struggling to breathe, since the condition can cause suffocation. Allergies affect the chest; throat and breathing cause a person to feel stuffy. Some of the problems that emerge from allergies include sneezing, coughing, watery eyes, running nose, aching head, and so on.

Asthma and allergies affect millions of people each year. The condition wakes them up during the night hours causing them to gag or grasp for air. Their breathing is often affected, which makes these people feel helpless.

Asthma alone can set up as pneumonia and can cause a person to grasp for air. Asthma affects the respiratory system, including the bronchial and pulmonary area. Asthma is a reversed disease that affects the lungs. This disease causes inflammation to attack the airway. The person will wheeze, struggle to breathe and so on. Asthma causes flare-ups, coughing, swelling, muscle tightness, mucus buildup, and so on.

When a person is diagnosed with asthma, it causes swelling, which creates shallow breathing. The person will breathe heavily and swiftly gasping for air.

Some people are born with asthma, which goes away as they mature. In many instances, the condition turns to allergies. Some people however continue life with asthmatic symptoms after birth and thereafter. Asthma may include mild symptoms, which develop into severe conditions. The condition is life threatening regardless. Asthma requires ongoing medical observation and treatment.

Allergies are affected millions of people each day, yet to find relief individual studies must take place. We are all different, so we have to find what works best for us.

Studies show however that yoga is a healing agent. When we practice yoga, we practice natural breathing. Natural breathing helps us to take control of our respiratory system, complete body and mind. To practice yoga however, you must have a will to take control of you. If you want, relief yoga is your answer. , You must continue visiting your doctor regularly to continue relief.

CHAPTER 4- TREATING ALLERGIES

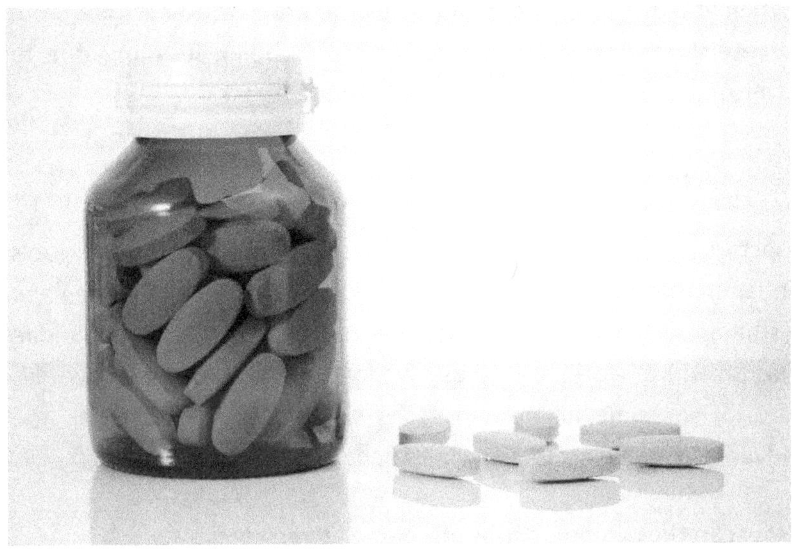

Recently, studies showed that the latest medications and over-the-counter remedies may be responsible for increasing allergies, asthma and other related disease.

Experts recently discovered that treatments are indefinable. One of the prime medications used to treat asthma however proved beneficial. The problem however is that most people who were prescribed these medications overused the product. It led to more problems. The medication included a bronchodilator. This is an inhaler, which has an albuterol and beta-based agonist medication to treat allergies and asthma. This medication was discovered to bring relief to those suffering with the disease.

Inhalers reopened the airways so that the patient could breathe freely. The inhaler quickly resolved mucus buildup. Doctors warned patients against overusing the drug, yet patients ignored the doctors warning. They found relief from this medication, and used it when it was not necessary. Now doctors are looking for other remedies to treat allergies and asthma.

How overusing inhalers affect you:

When you overuse inhalers it causes the problem to become more severe. In addition, the medication stops doing its thing due to overuse and it causes you to have frequent attacks.

How do doctors treat patients now?

Doctors often prescribe Corticosteroids. This medication cools inflammation that builds up from infections, such as allergies and asthma. Doctors often prescribe Prednisone. This medication alone has proven to work, as well as save lives. While this remedy works, it also has some highly dangerous side effects that showed too adverse in many instances when taking.

How can these medications affect me adversely?

Studies showed that these medications could cause damage to the bones. Glaucoma is affected in some instances. Studies showed that people gained weight while taking this medication, as well the hormones changed. Dependency was another problem found when taking this drug.

How can I find allergy relief, which doesn't have adverse effects on me?

Perhaps you want to consider yoga. Yoga is a natural workout that teaches you to breathe naturally. Acupuncture has proven to relieve symptoms stemming from allergies or asthma.

Diet, exercise, yoga and acupuncture may be the best solution when searching for allergy relief. The natural actions and nutrients will supply your body what it needs to live healthy. You should also practice avoidance. If you avoid the irritants that get to you, you can find allergy relief.

Products and how they can help you find relief:

Dehumidifiers and humidifiers are products that can help you find allergy relief. Some of the latest products designed by Hepa may be of interest to you. The filtration systems are designed to purify the air. Some of the impurities that cause asthma and allergy attacks include dust mites, dust, mold, mildew, pollen and so on. The irritants can cause major health conditions.

Mold and mildew alone will cause itchy eyes, swelling, rashes, and sniffles and so on. Mold and mildew are harsh and should be minimized to avoid allergy attacks and asthma.

Online you will find a nice line of products made by Hepa and other manufacturers. Keep in mind however; Hepa is designed to purify the air up to 95 percent or higher. This product will remove microns from the air, as well as other harmful irritants that cause allergy flare-ups and asthma attacks.

To find allergy relief you should also learn cleaning tips to avoid irritants. You want to learn how to rid your home of dust mites. Dust is something else you want to keep down. Mold and mildew cleaners are available, yet read the label so that you do not purchase chemicals that cause flare-ups. To learn more about allergy relief go online and read the information available to you.

Using Medications

More and more people are known to have allergies each day. It is a known fact that 1 in 4 Americans have allergies. With the high rate of known allergies, soon 50% of the US Citizens will be diagnosed with some type of allergy. Experts are struggling harder than ever to find cures so that people can continue living their normal lives.

Much different medication can be bought now to treat allergies. Your physician prescribes some medications and some can be purchased over-the-counter. Prescription medicine is being prescribed to more than 50% of the known allergy patients and 35% are taking over the counter.

Oral antihistamines are the most common medications that are being prescribed now. Most of the oral antihistamines will cause drowsiness and can be bought over-the-counter; there is also the non-drowsy but it has to be prescribed by a physician. Not all allergy patients get the full effect from the non-drowsy so they have to go back to the other one.

Oral antihistamines are not a permanent relief; short term only. When taking oral antihistamines read all warnings; this medication will react the same way as if you were to be picked up for OUIL or DUI. The oral treatment can cause drowsiness, and keep your brain from thinking and functioning in a normal way. Other side effects may include anxiety, nausea, and loss of appetite, dry mouth, and dizziness.

Doctors recommend Benadryl as a temporary quick fix because of its fast action until you can get in to see them. Benadryl is a good product to keep in the medicine cabinet for the relief of itching caused from poison ivy and oak, sunburns and insect bites as well as relieving the itching caused from allergies. Use with caution and read the side effects on the labels, not everyone can use Benadryl.

Antihistamines can be bought as a nasal spray also when prescribed by the doctor. Doctors seem to think that it increases the concentration where needed and help to relieve the allergy symptoms at the same time. Using the nasal spray helps to relieve the allergy symptoms up to 12 hours. There are side effects so be sure to read the warnings as you would any medication some of them are headaches, drowsiness, and has a bitter taste as it drips through the nasal passage.

Medication for the eyes comes in over-the-counter in a teardrop form. This is to wash out the eye to help relieve the redness and the antihistamines reduce the itching.

Prescribed medication for the eyes is given for different reasons. Antihistamine drops are prescribed for the redness, itching, and swelling in the eyes.

Nonsteroidal anti-inflammatory drops are given for the mast cell stabilizer effect to prevent the release of histamine. For the chronic symptoms like the itching and swelling Corticosteroids drops are given. As all medications be sure to consult your physician before using if you are not for certain what you need.

Decongestants come in oral and nasal sprays helping to relieve the allergy symptoms letting you have a better night of sleep. It opens the nasal passages so you are relieved from that stuffy nose feeling. Decongestants can be bought in pill form, sprays and liquids. Like all medications, there are side effects and warnings so are sure to read the label before using. Doctors advise that people who have heart disease, diabetes, and are taking certain antidepressants not to take decongestion sprays, liquids, etc.

You can find many allergy relief articles and methods for relieving allergy symptoms on the Internet and in books. Do some research and talk to your doctor about getting relief to a more normal life. Learning about herbs can help you find allergy relief.

Herbal Treatments

Taking treatment with herbs is the all-natural way to stay healthy. Remember when taking herbs even though they are considered safe, that some of them may counteract with your prescribed medications. So, be sure to read and learn about the herbs you are interested in taking to avoid problems. If you do not understand what you are reading and taking, consult with your doctor before starting anything new.

Some of the herbs that are being used today used for allergy treatment are Marshmallow root to help relieve mucous from the body. Burdock is used to clear the congestion in the respiratory system. To sooth, the throat and clear congestion, try using Mullein and to getting the antibiotic effect use Goldenseal Root it contains antibacterial and anti-fungal.

Eye Bright is a very effective natural herb to help the allergies by helping the congestion and hay fever that you might be experiencing. A natural antihistamine for allergies and fights infection use Capsicum. Stinging nettle is used to treat hay fever and another natural for the allergy treatments you're looking for.

Vitamin C and natural anti-histamine is found in Acerola Cherry. Rosemary is a good anti-inflammatory and strengthens the nervous system too. For reducing mucus and chest congestion, try White Pine.

Using herbs are just one way to help relieve allergy symptoms. Allergies can be deadly to a person if they are having chronic problems and do not get relief fast. When a person is having an allergy attack, they start to have a hard time breathing they can hyperventilate, and the oxygen level will go down. Remember herbs are not a cure they only help to relieve the symptoms. Consult a doctor if the symptoms do not seem to get better.

Other way to help is your home environment is very important to someone that has allergies. The home needs to be kept clean from dust, pollen and mold as much as possible. Do some research on items that can be bought for keeping the home free from dust, pollen and mold? You could be saving someone's life.

Keep the home clean by vacuuming 2 or 3 times a week. Dust mites like to live in dark places and where there is moisture. Have a good filter on your sweeper to catch the flying dust before it has a chance to escape.

TV's, stereos, furniture and carpets are just a few of the dust mites' favorite places to multiply. Be sure that you clean behinds these things and spray the carpets and furniture.

There is also a carpet shampoo to help get rid of the dust mites imbedded into the carpet and furniture. Keeping the beds free from dust mites is another thing. Encase your box springs, mattress and pillows with a zippered casing to keep the dust from bedding into them.

Check out the basement. Mold lives in damp areas and most basements are damp in need of a dehumidifier. Dehumidifiers can be bought at most hardware and department stores. Be sure that it is equipped with a filter on it to cash the dust down there along with drawing out the moisture that can cause the mold. You can purchase a cleaner to help clean up the mold that may have already started growing in your basement.

Having allergies is no fun and helping you or your loved one to be able to live a more normal life is very important. Unveiling the causes behind allergy relief can help you avoid attacks.

Can Vinegar Help?

Chemicals can affect us in many ways. Some cleaners we use have harmful chemicals that can kill us if inhaled, or digested. We need to learn how to clean our home to avoid irritants that cause allergies. To get started we need to consider chemicals.

How vinegar works:

Vinegar is distilled. It's made of grains and acidity products that come from natural sources. Vinegar has a strong aroma that sways most people from using the product, yet if you were to clean your home with vinegar, the irritants will stay away also. They too hate the nasty aroma that comes from vinegar.

Most chemicals we use for cleaning have hasty elements that interrupt the respiratory system, bronchia and sinuses. If we are to find allergy relief, we must convert to a new way of living. This means we should only use natural products to clean our home.

Lysol is a common household cleaning product. Many people use this product, yet some people suffer severe headaches after spraying the chemicals. Lysol has an active ingredient known as dimethylbenzylammonium chloride, which is said to eliminate germs.

The chemicals in Lysol are far less hazardous than other chemicals according to experts. Yet, the chemicals when overexposed to are toxic. The toxics are linked to birth defects, cancers, and have been linked to allergy attacks.

One thing for sure, many household cleaning products contain toxics. Not anything toxic surely should be worth letting into our environment. Most of your air fresheners, soaps, bleaches, shampoos, antiperspirant, hair spray, cleansers, detergents, and paint thinners and so on are toxic.

Still we have to clean our homes. Instead of using chemicals with harmful toxics, take your cleaning journey to organic reserves.

Vinegar is great for removing stains. Vinegar will keep away irritants. You can also use natural products made by SFI products. Most of these products are safe to use. In fact, thousands of people have tried these products and have giving good reports. Go online to check reviews before considering the product. The vendors enable you to make money from selling the products as well. For the most part, you want to think health, so consider what you need to find allergy relief.

Filters for vacuums should be considered also when searching for allergy relief. High-efficient filters can reduce irritants from you home over 90%. Hepa manufactured by NASA is one of the best filters on the market. This product was intended for use in plants, yet it was approved by proper channels and is now used in homes, hospitals and so on.

Cleaning beds and furniture is important. If you want to keep, dust mites and dust at bay wash your bedding weekly in hot water. You may want to add vinegar to your wash to help fight dust mites and dust.

Studies show that furniture made of upholstery has higher potentials of causing dust and dust mites to stick. If possible, you may want to invest in foam-packed furniture.

Wood collects dust. Televisions and carpets collect dust also. It is wise to cleanse the areas frequently. Dust at least once each day. To clean wood tries using the oils instead of the sprays. Oils are healthy for breathing than sprays.

If you have pets in your home, keep in mind that most allergies emerge from pet dander. If you are not prepared to separate from your friend, then take more time to clean your home. If you clean your home each day, you can keep irritants at bay. Perhaps you can designate one area of your home to your pet only. Clean air in the home is the start to allergy relief.

CHAPTER 5- NUTS – SMALL BUT DEADLY TO SOME

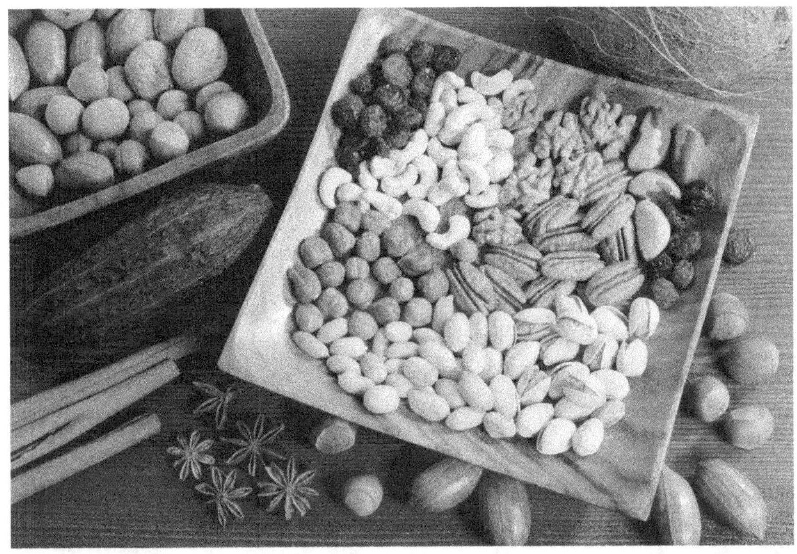

All available statistics indicate that the food allergy most widely suffered by the greatest number of people in the West is to peanuts. It is, therefore, important to understand what peanuts are, and more importantly, what they are not.

A peanut is distinct from tree based nuts, in that it is a legume rather than a true nut. It is a close relative of the soy bean, kidney bean, garden pea and lentil. Such plants carry nitrogen fixing bacteria on their roots, and, as a result, they add extra nitrogen to the soil in which they grow. This enriches the soil, and it is for this reason that such plants are extremely popular with farmers as crops. A tree nut, on the other hand, is generally the dried fruit of that tree, and while tree nut allergy is every bit as severe as peanut allergy, it is far less common.

Because they are entirely different, it is possible that people can be allergic to peanuts while they are perfectly okay with tree nuts, and vice versa. However, for some reason that is not yet fully understood, there does seem to be some correlation between peanut and tree nut allergies.

While there appears to be no particular reason why a peanut allergy sufferer should be more susceptible to having the same problem with tree nuts than anyone else, a high percentage of peanut allergy sufferers also suffer adverse effects when they consume tree nuts. It has also been established that children who suffer a peanut allergy are more likely to suffer other food allergies, including tree nuts, in adulthood. There does, therefore, appear to be some connection between the two, probably because of a general weakening of a food allergy sufferer's immune system.

In the USA alone, it is believed that up to i.5 million people may be allergic to peanuts. While the USA is a major producer and consumer of peanut based foodstuffs, this picture is broadly mirrored in other major Western civilizations. According to the Asthma and Allergy Foundation of America, an allergic reaction to peanut consumption is the largest food related cause of death in the USA.

In numerical terms, based on statistics produced by the Food Allergy & Anaphylaxis Network, around 100 people will die every year in the USA as a result of an adverse reaction to peanuts. This is out of a total of approximately 150 people who die every year from an allergic reaction to foods, so peanut allergy is clearly the most serious food allergy in the USA.

The same advisory group believes that an adverse reaction to peanuts is responsible for 15,000 emergency room visits every year as well. While approximately 0.5% of adults and children have a peanut allergy in the USA, approximately 25% of children who are afflicted by this condition will grow out of it in their teens or early adulthood.

Understanding the Basics of Peanut Allergy

An allergy to peanuts is a condition which afflicts the immune system of the body, where your body will suffer from a wide range of symptoms following exposure to some of the proteins in peanuts. Peanut allergy is the most prevalent food allergy in the USA, and for many people, even the minutest amount of peanut-based material in their food can trigger a dangerous and sometimes fatal allergic reaction.

In fact, peanut allergy is the most common food allergy in almost every Western country, although it is extremely rare in the people of Asian and Oriental societies, places where peanuts form a far more important part of the indigenous diet. Because of its prevalence in the West, however, it is essential to appreciate that it only needs the tiniest exposure to peanut-based proteins to trigger a severe allergic reaction in some people. For instance, those who are most sensitive to peanut-based proteins can suffer a serious reaction to as little as 2 mg of such protein.

As a peanut contains around 200 mg protein, this means that such a person will react to anything that contains as little as 1% of a peanut! Indeed, as evidence of this, you need look no further than this headline taken from 'The Times' newspaper in the UK:

'Death from chip dipped in curry'

An otherwise healthy young woman in her early 20s with a severe peanut allergy and asthma simply dipped her chip (French fry) into a sauce in a restaurant, and died in the ambulance on the way to hospital as a direct result of doing so.

How Serious Is It?

An allergic reaction to peanut protein is likely to be the most deadly allergic reaction, as it accounts for four out of every five life threatening occurrences of anaphylactic shock in both the UK and the USA. While it is relatively rare that the peanut allergen will kill you (15,000 people visit emergency rooms as a result of their peanut allergy, but only 100 die every year, so the numbers are on your side!), it is nevertheless extremely dangerous and the effects of peanut allergy can be extremely unpleasant.

Anaphylaxis and Anaphylactic Shock

Anaphylaxis is the word used to define a severe, extreme and rapid allergic reaction that most commonly involves more than one part of the body. In the most extreme circumstances, anaphylaxis is fatal. The word anaphylaxis itself was coined by scientists who were attempting to immunize animals from poison by injecting them with a small dose of that same poison. In their experiments, the animals invariably died! However, this process of stimulating an immune condition by using a small dose of the same chemical, which is known as 'prophylaxis', had been used with great success for many years. The scientists concerned therefore created the term 'anaphylaxis' to suggest a situation where even the smallest dosage of a chemical being introduced to the body could create an extreme adverse physical reaction.

Anaphylaxis is a reference to the opposite of the protection offered by prophylaxis. As far as current scientific thinking is concerned, the word anaphylaxis refers to any allergic reaction, irrespective of how serious it is. For medical doctors and allergy specialists, however, the term is far more commonly used to describe a severe allergic reaction.

Anaphylaxis might be a potentially life-threatening occurrence if the symptoms include:

•A struggle for breath;

•Moderate to serious stomach or abdominal pain;

•Having difficulty swallowing;

•Vomiting or nausea;

•Hives;

•Diarrhea.

To take this one stage further, an anaphylactic shock is the most severe form of anaphylactic allergic reaction, and it requires immediate medical attention, primarily because it can cause the bronchial tissues of the lungs to expand, which will restrict the sufferer's ability to breathe.

At the same time, bodily extremities begin to turn blue, and the face and neck can begin to swell. In this condition, the sufferer's blood pressure can drop alarmingly and suddenly, and if the condition is not treated, it can lead to death within as little as 10 minutes from the onset of the allergic attack. However, as long as the patient is in a position where they can receive immediate medical attention, a shot of epinephrine (adrenaline) can be administered to the patient. This will reverse most of the most serious symptoms of anaphylactic shock, and the patient should return to normal quickly.

It is nowadays increasingly common that, once a serious peanut allergy has been diagnosed, patients will be given auto injectors with which to administer their own dose of adrenaline when a serious allergic reaction begins to set in. Nevertheless, the importance of seeking immediate medical attention for anyone suffering anaphylactic shock cannot be overestimated, because at the present time, epinephrine is the only proven reliable treatment for anaphylaxis.

Anaphylaxis and Biphasic Reaction

One important aspect of anaphylaxis and anaphylactic shock that many people who do not suffer from food allergies do not understand is that as many as 30% of sufferers will undergo a biphasic reaction to their anaphylaxis. What this means is that, without any further exposure to the peanut proteins that caused their condition in the first place, they can suffer a further allergic reaction which can in some cases be every bit as severe or serious as the first reaction. This can occur anything from one hour to eight hours after the original reaction, and this means two things.

Firstly, it is absolutely imperative that anyone who is looking after someone who has suffered an anaphylactic shock as a result of exposure to the proteins in peanuts should keep a very close eye on that person for several hours afterwards.

As three out of every 10 food allergy sufferers can suffer biphasic attacks, the chances of the allergic reaction coming back without any further stimulus or warning cannot be ignored. Secondly, the biphasic nature of anaphylactic reactions to even the minutest trace of the proteins from peanuts makes a peanut allergy one of the most dangerous of all food allergies.

Other Signs and Symptoms

Not every person who has an allergy to peanuts is going to suffer an anaphylactic shock. Indeed, in the majority of cases, the people that do so are most likely to be those who are otherwise hypersensitive and therefore tend to suffer the most extreme reactions. Most people will suffer far milder allergic reactions to peanut proteins, but despite this, these reactions will differ and vary in severity from person to person.

The most common symptoms of an allergic reaction to peanut protein might include any of the following, occurring just minutes, up to an hour, after consumption of the offending foodstuff:

•Itchy eyes;

•Stomach ache and/or nausea;

•Tingling lips or tongue;

•Hives;

•Itchy skin rash;

•Runny nose.

After the initial onset of these symptoms, they may well lessen for anyone whose allergic condition is not too serious. On the other hand, for someone who has a severe allergic condition, these symptoms are more likely to worsen, and could then include:

•Tight throat and labored breathing;

•Coughing, wheezing and choking;

•Extreme nausea and/or vomiting;

•Diarrhea.

With the onset of any of these symptoms, medical help should be sought as quickly as possible, or a dose of adrenaline should be administered as appropriate.

CHAPTER 6- THE ORIGINS OF PEANUT ALLERGY

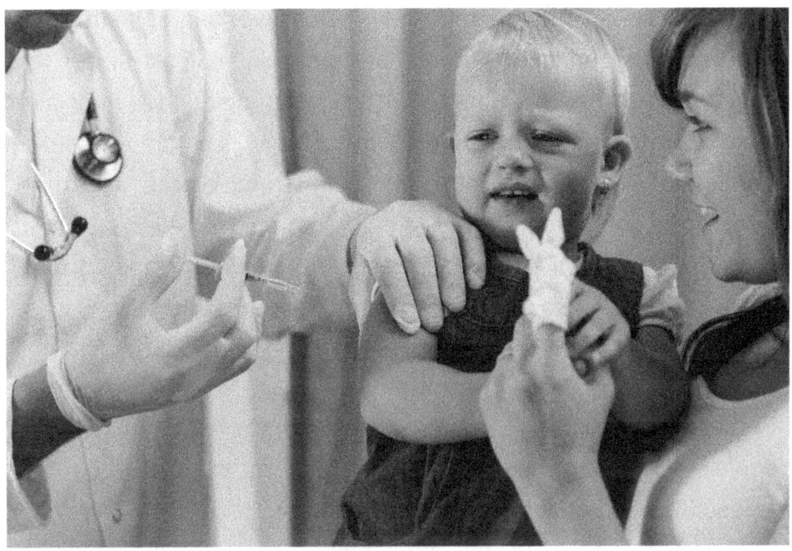

An allergic reaction to the proteins in peanuts is unlikely to happen the very first time you consume those proteins. Indeed, the first time you eat peanuts, for example, it is extremely unlikely that you will suffer any kind of adverse reaction, and you will, most probably, thoroughly enjoy eating them! When you do so, however, the immune system of your body will begin to develop antibodies to the proteins in those peanuts.

A similar thing can happen if you eat foods that have been cooked in incompletely processed peanut oil. These antibodies are called immunoglobulin E (IgE), and what they are going to do in the future is recognize the peanut proteins that you consume as an unwanted invading enemy. The next time you consume peanuts or any foodstuff that contains the proteins from them, your body will recognize the proteins, and the IgE antibodies that your immune system previously developed will attack them. You are now suffering an allergic reaction. This reaction comes about because the IgE antibodies cause certain chemicals to be released into the body, one of which is histamine.

Histamine can adversely affect the efficient working of a sufferer's respiratory system, cardiovascular system, skin and gastrointestinal tract. Therefore, when you are suffering an allergic reaction as a result of consuming peanut proteins, you will commonly suffer shortness of breath, wheezing, vomiting, stomach ache and so on. It is reasonable to ask why this should happen. However, scientists have not so far been able to ascertain why peanut proteins should induce some people's bodies to create antibodies in this way, while it does not do so for the majority.

In other words, at the moment, science cannot tell you why some people will develop a peanut allergy, while most will not. For this reason, it is impossible to predict with any degree of certainty whether any particular individual child or adult will develop a peanut allergy. However, it is possible to have some idea of children who are more likely than others to develop an allergy to the proteins in peanuts by looking at the medical history of their parents, and in particular at whether either of them has suffered an allergy at any time so far.

If one parent has suffered from any kind of allergy themselves (and, note, this is any form of allergy, and not specifically limited to an allergic reaction to peanuts, or, indeed to any food allergy), then the chances of their child also suffering from an allergy are 50% higher than that of a child of parents neither of whom have ever suffered an allergy. If, however, both parents have suffered from allergies at any time in their lives, then the chances of their offspring doing so increase to 70% on the same basis.

It can be seen from this that, while science has still not come up with a definite answer as to why some people seem more prone to allergies than others, there does seem to be a hereditary factor involved. In the majority of cases, when a child is going to develop an allergy of any form, they will start to do so at a very young age.

Once they have developed this allergy, then for around three in every four, this will be a lifetime condition, whereas for the other one in four, they will grow out of it as they move into their teens and early adulthood.

Peanut Allergy versus Intolerance

Some people are intolerant to peanuts and peanut-based foodstuffs. On eating them, they will suffer minor stomach upsets, temporary vomiting and perhaps even a bout of diarrhea. This is not the same, however, as an outright allergic reaction to peanuts, because then the immune system of the sufferer is not attacking the peanut proteins with antibodies.

All that this is happening is that the person involved might find that peanuts are simply too rich for their metabolism, and they will suffer a mildly unpleasant reaction as a result. Alternatively, some people will find peanuts (and, indeed, any foodstuff coming from or based on legumes) difficult to digest, and they might suffer indigestion or mild stomach pains as a direct result of this. However, these are not allergic reactions, as the body is not 'on the attack' in this scenario.

How Peanut Proteins Enter Your Body

The most direct way for anyone to take in peanuts or anything derived from them is by eating foodstuffs which contain them. Similarly, consuming foodstuffs that have been cooked in incompletely processed peanut oil is also a direct and straightforward consumption of the proteins in peanuts that cause allergic reactions.

In the case of oil, be particularly wary of gourmet or hand pressed peanut oils. In addition to such types of peanut protein consumption, however, it is also possible to take in traces of peanut proteins if they come into contact with the skin or the lips. Here, the antibodies created by your immune system are every bit as likely to attack these proteins as they would be if you had eaten a peanut butter sandwich! However, coming into direct contact with the proteins from peanuts that cause severe allergic reactions is entirely preventable as long as you remain diligent and careful.

It is important to understand that there are other ways that you can come into contact with peanut proteins which are far more difficult to prevent.

From cross-contact

Cross contact exposure to the proteins that cause allergic reactions will almost always come about completely accidentally. For example, if a foodstuff company that processes peanuts uses exactly the same machines to process other non-peanut related foodstuffs, then crosses contact 'contamination' of the non-peanut related foodstuffs can occur when that machinery is not cleaned thoroughly. While in most developed countries this is becoming less likely to happen as food hygiene rules and regulations become ever tighter, it is still not impossible, and when it does, there is very little that one can do about this kind of exposure to peanuts based proteins.

Be on the lookout for cross-contact contamination possibilities in the home or in everyday life as well. For example, using the same knives and food chopping or preparation area for foods that might contain peanut extracts and those that you yourself eat is a recipe for disaster. Likewise, if other people have used a knife to make a peanut butter sandwich, do not be tempted to use it after them without washing it thoroughly first.

Watch out when you are frequenting common food areas like ice cream parlors as well. Such places commonly use the same scoop for several types of ice cream and, unless you know for a fact that they are scrupulously clean, you could be taking a big risk of cross-contact contamination.

Through inhalation

Some aerosol sprays contain peanut extracts, and for any sufferer from a peanut allergy, being in the same room as someone using such a spray could trigger an allergic reaction. If someone is using peanut flour for cooking, then microscopically small amounts of that flour can be released into the surrounding air, and become airborne as a direct result. Inhaling these microscopic traces of peanut flour could trigger an allergic reaction in anyone who suffers from a severe allergy to peanuts. Finally, avoid anyone who is using a peanut cooking oil spraying device, because this will again release microscopically small traces of oil into the air. Anyone who breathes any of those oil traces who suffers from a peanut allergy may suffer a reaction because of doing so.

Avoid More Than Just the Peanuts

It is extremely important that anyone who suffers from a peanut allergy understands that there are certain foods that they must stay away from in order to avoid exacerbating their condition. While it is always important that you educate yourself as to what these foods are, you should also learn to read and understand food packaging labels and the ingredients that those foods contain. It does not stop there, however.

You must, for example, be extremely vigilant and careful about oils or creams that you apply to your skin, because it is possible that traces of peanut proteins can get into your bloodstream in this way. No matter how careful you are, it is virtually impossible to guarantee that you never come into contact with any foodstuff or products that contain traces of peanut proteins, but you must always be on your guard. You must also be willing to take the time and make the effort to read the labels and ingredient lists on everything that you ever eat, cook with or rub on your skin.

On the following couple of pages, you will see a list of foodstuffs that you must avoid if you have a peanut allergy. Some of these are obvious, while others are perhaps less so, but they can all contain peanut protein and eating them will, therefore, expose you to a risk of allergic reaction. You will note that peanut oil is not included on this list, while it has already been mentioned on two or three occasions in this book.

This is because completely pure peanut oil has all of the harmful proteins removed from it during the purifying process. However, lots of the peanut oil that is commercially manufactured and bought from supermarkets and hypermarkets is not completely purified, and it will therefore still contain trace elements of the proteins that anyone with a peanut allergy needs to avoid. For that reason, while peanut oil is not included on this list, you should nevertheless avoid eating foods that are cooked using it.

Also, do not make the mistake of thinking that, because a particular foodstuff is not included in this list it will be safe for you to eat. New food products come onto the market almost every day, while some of those that have been around for some time regularly undergo changes to the manufacturing process. Furthermore, the diet that you eat everyday will, to a certain extent, the dictated by where you live, because while some products are available internationally, many others are only available in their country of original manufacture.

For all these reasons, it is impossible to produce a comprehensive list of every foodstuff that might contain peanut proteins that covers the whole world! While the following list covers many of the most common foodstuffs that contain peanuts and/or peanut extracts, the simplest answer is always going to be, if you are in any doubt about eating something – anything – do not do it!

Peanuts are used in many dried, bottled or canned processed foods as a thickening or emulsifying agent. In addition, pre-prepared food and fried pre-prepared foods, including such dietary staples as roasted chicken, may also include peanuts as a flavor enhancer. On top of that, all of the following can contain peanuts or peanut byproducts in which traces of the protein that cause an allergic reaction can still be found. If you are thinking of eating any of these, you should ensure that you check and double check the label before doing so.

Common foods to avoid

•Peanut butter;

•Peanut flour;

•Sunflower seeds;

•Granola;

•Commercially produced breakfast cereals;

•Mixed nut products;

•Salad dressing;

•Energy bars;

•Whole or full grain bread;

•Store baked biscuits or cookies;

•Baking mixes;

•Sauces (peanuts are often used as a thickening agent);

•Soups (especially dried soup mixes);

•Egg rolls;

•Ice cream;

•Pesto;

•Satay sauces;

•Chocolate ice cream;

•Nutella spread;

•Vegetarian burgers and burger mixes;

•Nougat;

•Marzipan.

As suggested above, although pure peanut oil commonly has all of the harmful proteins processed out of it, other cooking oils such as those marketed as 'Groundnut Oil' will have the proteins largely left intact because they add extra flavor to the oil, and therefore to the food that is cooked in it. For that reason, they are to be avoided.

CHAPTER 7- FOOD LABELS AND YOUR IMMUNITY

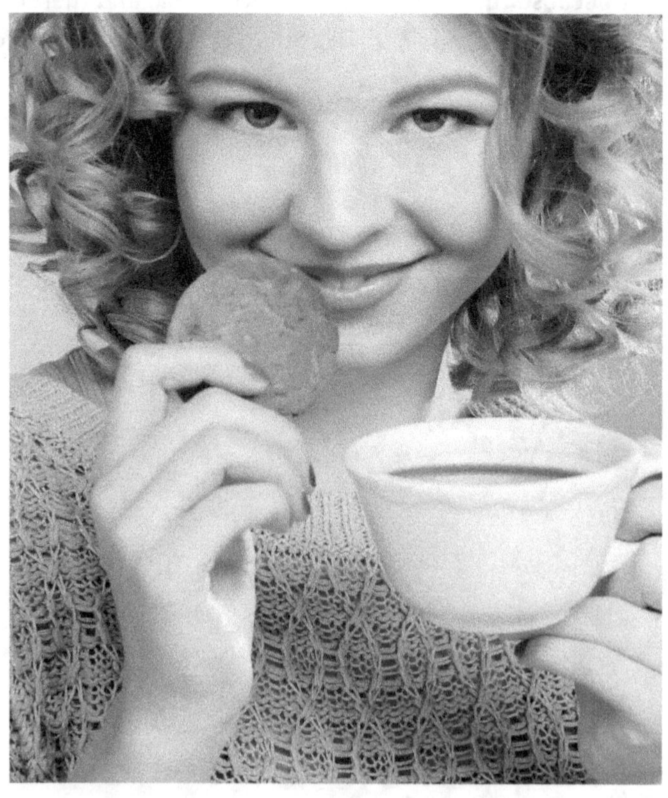

Because the general awareness of the seriousness of peanut allergy sufferers consuming peanuts has improved in leaps and bounds over the past few years, food labeling standards have also improved immeasurably.

Food labeling standards are becoming more uniform and standardized on a global basis as well. The international organization that controls matters such as food labeling and global standardization is the Codex Committee on Food Labelling (CCFL), which was originally founded in 1963, and now boasts 72 member nations, in addition to the European Union and 27 international organizations, as members. The CCFL has done much over the years to ensure that the ingredients that could potentially harm consumers are always clearly marked on the label, so that it is now almost universally accepted that any products that contain peanuts or peanut protein should be marked as such.

It is not always specifically necessary that peanuts are mentioned on food labels by name, however. For this reason, be on the lookout for 'alternative' label descriptions that might suggest or imply that there could be peanuts in the food that you are investigating, such as:

•'may contain peanuts/nuts'

•'produced on equipment shared with nuts or peanuts'

•'produced in a facility that also processes peanuts/nuts' .As long as consumers are willing to read the labels, it is almost impossible to eat or consume any product that contains peanuts by accident. It is therefore surprising that the incidence of peanut allergies has shown a sharp increase over the last 5 to 10 years, not only in the USA, but also in Australia and the UK as well. One theory as to why this is happening is that children are being introduced to peanuts and products that contain peanut matter at a younger age. Given that peanut byproducts are still commonly used in the manufacture of candy in many countries, this may be a valid point.

Another theory suggests that because processed soy byproducts are nowadays used in commercially available baby milk formulas, this encourages the immune systems of even the youngest babies to start producing antibodies at an extremely young age. From there, it might only be a small step to a point where those antibodies are used to defend the body against peanut protein; hence soy byproducts are doing the groundwork that allows a peanut allergy to develop a little later.

Perhaps the most interesting theory is that modern man has a less effective and combative immune system, due to our increasing use of antibiotics, vaccinations and fewer impurities in our foodstuff because of improved food processing procedures. Whatever the reason, peanut allergies in children are becoming increasingly common, and that represents a worrying trend.

Dining Out Could Be Serious

Although not politically correct to use the terminology nowadays, there was a time when those who suffered from a peanut allergy were said to have 'Chinese restaurant syndrome'. This is because while peanuts are not widely used in Western cuisine, across the whole of Asia and the East, peanuts are an essential ingredient of a huge range of dishes and cooking styles. For this reason, whenever eating in an Asian or Oriental restaurant, it is a reasonable assumption that peanuts will have been used in many of the dishes on the menu.

While a large number of restaurants will highlight the dishes that are made with peanuts (or sometimes tree nuts) on the menu, it is not safe to assume that they all will. While peanut allergies are increasingly common in many Western countries, it is rare to hear of people in Eastern countries who suffer from a peanut allergy. This is partially as a result of the propensity to use peanuts in almost every principle style of cuisine across Asia, so that people have been used to eating peanut-based foodstuffs over many generations and hundreds of years.

Their digestive systems have long since got used to dealing with peanuts and peanut proteins. This does, however, have one negative side-effect as far as a Western restaurant-goer is concerned. Because many restaurants owners and workers have never suffered any problems with peanuts themselves, nor have they ever met any compatriots who have, mentioning that a particular dish contains peanuts might seem irrelevant.

Always ask, and try to address your question to someone who knows what they are talking about, like the manager or the chef. If you're still left in any doubt, then the simple answer is to take no chances. If you are not certain what are in it, do not be tempted to eat it, no matter how good it looks!

CHAPTER 8- MOLDS AND ALLERGIES

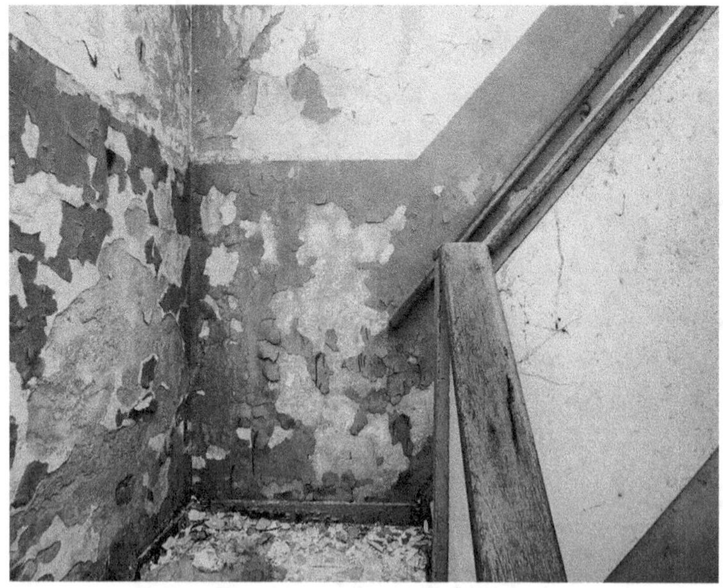

Did you know that you could get allergies from mold?

Mold is everywhere, including inside your home as well as outside. Many people are allergic to mold. Therefore, you need to try to prevent mold from entering your home as much as possible. Mold usually develops in damp areas.

There are various types of molds around and every kind can affect you in a negative way. Mold is also air born so that it can be hard to find in your home.

Mold can get in your nose and build up. You may not know until it attacks your respiratory and bronchial system.

Where does mold hide?

Mold is normally found in many places where dampness is found. Such places like your shower stall, your basement, or a closet, even in the refrigerator in the fresh food drawer mold will hide. Mold can develop in your trashcan, or even in the laundry room.

Mold is outside. Mold grows on trees, even the ground. Sometimes, you see it growing on your home. Mold is all from the dampness outside. When it grows in your home its cause from too much moister so you may want to watch how damp it gets in your home to help to count down the growth of the mold.

How would I know if I were allergic to mold?

If you had allergies, I believe that you would know but in some cases, you would not. Here are some things that you might want to look for. These are only the common symptoms that are associated with mold.

Nasal stuffiness, eye irritation, wheezing, cold or the flu like symptoms, could be a rash, fever, shortness of breath, fatigue, sometime even lung infection. Most of the time, these symptoms do not just go away it takes a long time to get rid of them. If this happened to you, you need to go see your family doctor before it gets worse.

What food has mold in it?

Some food contains a lot of mold so if you have any kind of allergies to mold you need to stay away from this food. Like things that have yeast in it for example, bread. Beer, wine, mushrooms, dried fruit, soy sauce, vinegar, mayonnaise other dressing, catsup, pickled things like picked beets, green sour cream as well as cheese can develop mold. To prevent from have an allergy reaction you might want to monitor these foods, looking for mold.

How do I get rid of the mold in my home?

To get rid of the mold in your house you can use some beach and water. Wash the area with bleach. Bleach kills the mold.

Humidity in your home should be kept at a reasonable volume to avoid mold. Keep the humidity in all closed areas at a level.

You might want to take time and dry the shower stalls when you are done, make sure that things that may sweat are also dry. This will stop the mold from growing in your house around your toilet or bathroom.

Mold is the second poor airborne allergies, pollen being the first.

To avoid pollen and mold you will need to learn more cleaning tactics. For the most part, if you keep your home dry you can avoid mold.

Mold will also build up if the walls are moist. Some homes have moisture inside the walls. In this instance, black, orange, white and gray mold will often grow in the home. In this instance, you may need to hire a contractor or someone that specializes in home repair, etc. to resolve the problem. Find help today.

CHAPTER 9- FINDING RELIEF FROM POLLEN ALLERGIES

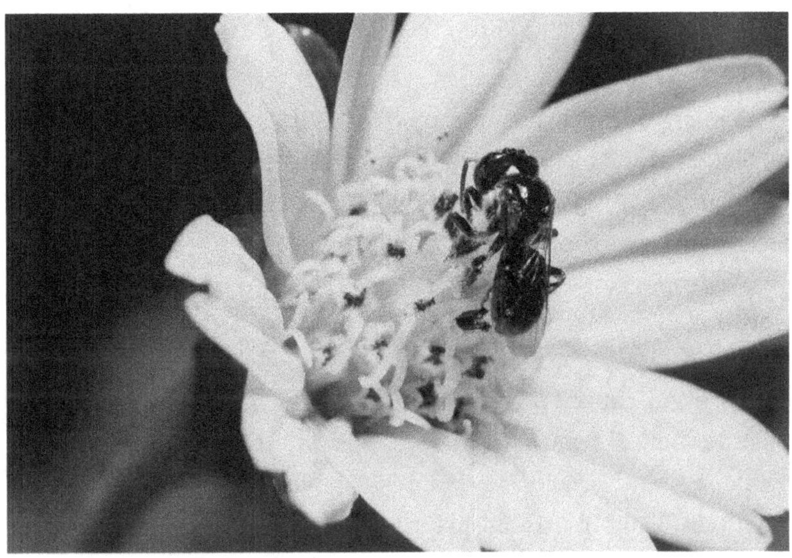

Today in my area, the high for pollen is 49 percent. This means that everyone around my area allergic to pollen will endure coughing, sneezing, watery eyes and so on. Some type of allergic reaction will occur in many homes, thus these people need to consider what they can do to find allergy relief while controlling pollen.

How to control pollen:

You can eliminate airborne irritants in the air. Place allergy-based pillow coverings over your bed pillows and then add your case. Commonly people endure hay fever, which is a seasonal reversible condition when pollen count is high. One of the common accounts of attacks stem from Rhinitis.

Rhinitis, like hay fever causes a person irritation, such as sneezing, coughing, itchy and watery eyes, dry throat, dry mouth and nose, and so on. The nose will often run and feel stuffy in many instances.

Rhinitis and hay fever can cause headaches, wheezing, and irritation. The condition can start insomnia, depression and weigh loss.

How can I control pollen?

In the air, outdoor pollen circulates. We have no control over pollen in natural air, yet we do have control of pollen in our homes. We can add a high-efficient air filter to our bedroom and other areas around the home to control pollen.

How pollen develops:

Pollen often causes seasonal allergies, which ordinarily is named Rhinitis. Pollen comes from weed, grass, trees and plants. The "male genetic" materials produce pollen from these natural resources. Units that hold male genetics are known as grain and have two surrounding walls to protect the grain. The intine is the deepest region of the grain that has thinning, delicate components.

The eternal walls are the exine, which has a high-tolerance to damage and is often thick. Pollination occurs when "pollen grains" are transferred. The plants transfer pollen grains from anthers and to male counterparts or organs. The male then transfers to stigma, which are the female counterparts.

After transferring is completed, fertilization begins. The pollen must go airborne to cause allergy reactions.

Pollen makes up cereals, grains, weeds, grass and so on. The pollen produces from these natural elements in nature. Cereal pollen usually causes fewer reactions than weeds. Since weeds typically release higher volumes of pollens into the air, it causes episodes of allergic reactions for people in all areas of the world. Pollen typically causes Rhinitis.

The common weeds that affect people causing allergy attacks include ragweed, buckhorn plantain, redroot pigweed, nettle, Western water hemps, sheep sorrel, thistle, lamp quarter and the burning bushes.

What areas pollen usually attacks include Northern America and the Western Hemispheres.

The time pollen hits your area:

During early spring pollen usually hits around February and up to March. Pollen hits late spring around April and throughout June and July. During summer months pollen hits around June and carries on to August.

Ragweed grows in fall. Some areas are isolated from pollen during winter months, yet in some areas such as South parts of California, Florida and Texas, ragweed will grow in the wintry months.

Do all pollens cause allergies?

In most instances, people are allergic to one type of pollen or the other, yet other pollen allergies can develop.

As you can see pollen is an outdoor, irritant that affects millions of people around the world. To control pollen you should learn what areas produce higher-volumes of pollination and in what months. During this time, you want to stay free of the outdoor areas where pollen circulates into the air.

If you live in Northern parts of America, during pollen season avoid outdoor areas where ragweed or similar weeds grow. Do you have seasonal allergies that call for relief?

Chapter 10- Seasonal and Psychical Allergies

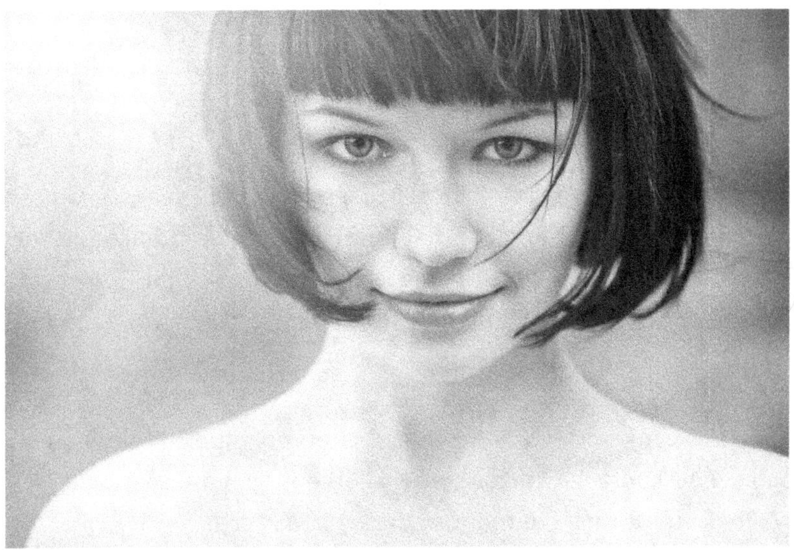

Seasonal allergies often include hay fever, Rhinitis and so on. Seasonal allergies often affect people at particular times of the year and it is caused from exposure to substances in the air. Airborne substances, such as pollen cause seasonal allergies, which doctors dub as Rhinitis or hay fever.

Usually seasonal allergies affect people during early and late spring and continue to affect people in the summer and fall months.

How do the symptoms start?

It depends on the person, but most people experience irritation at the membranes that line the nose. The allergic reaction causes Rhinitis to develop, which affects the lining of the membranes around the eyelids. The conjunctiva is affected as well, which is the white covering of the eyes. This can set in conjunctivitis and often Rhinitis. Still, other illnesses can cause such conditions to emerge.

How does hay fever develop?

Pollen usually triggers allergic reactions. Usually grass and pollinated weeds and so forth will cause hay fever to develop.

Trees pollinate, which include the birch, elm, oak, alder, juniper, maple, sagebrush, olive, and so on.

Seasonal allergies affect millions of people each year, yet most people are misled. The fact is hay fever can hit you throughout the year, yet it depends on the area you live. In addition, hay fever, Rhinitis and other conditions can develop especially if your immune system is sensitive to mold spores.

To avoid conjunctivitis and other related conditions you want to avoid eye contact with airborne allergens. If you have allergies wear glasses during the months, that pollen is high.

Many people allergic to seasonal allergens often endure asthma. While you may not know it asthma symptoms can develop, which include wheezing. If you have allergic reactions, it is wise to visit your doctor and explain in detail what symptoms you endure. This will help your doctor discover a diagnostic that follows proper treatment. Allergies can become life threatening so never take advantage of seasonal or other allergies believing that it is temporary.

What else you should know:

Conjunctivitis can develop into "Atopic Keratoconjunctivitis." This condition can cause blindness. The condition attacks everyone in all age groups but the prime targets are those over 30.

How can someone tell if they have Atopic Keratoconjunctivitis?

The symptoms are something you want to consider. If you experience blurring vision, your eyes burn, itch etc. and if you notice mucous discharging from your eyes, you may have Atopic Keratoconjunctivitis. If your eyes feel sensitive to sunlight followed by the named symptoms, see your doctor immediately.

How do doctors treat seasonal allergic reactions?

It depends on the allergy and the person. Doctors typically prescribe medications if the condition is mild. Rhinitis is often treated with antihistamines. In some instances when the patient does not have high or low blood pressure the doctor will prescribe decongestants. Pseudoephedrine is a common medicine doctors prescribe, which is a decongestant.

Should I seek medical help immediately if I notice mild allergic reactions?

If you are an allergist and know what you are doing you can take your own advice if you feel confident. You can use over-the-counter medications otherwise for a couple of days to see if it takes care of the problem. To answer your question however, logic should tell you to seek medical advice. Once more allergies can turn fatal. Do you have year-round allergies?

Physical Allergies

Physical allergies is commonly referred to for its name because if differs from most allergies. This condition is marked by reactions to physical stimulus that triggers the immune system.

What causes this condition?

Emotional stress, heat, cold air, sunlight, sweating, exercise, minor injuries, vibrations and similar responses are all responsible for physical allergies. The theory of the cause is that the protein changes in the skin and the immune system attacks it thinking it is a foreign object.

Some people are sensitive to the cold because of the abnormal protein in their blood indicating a serious condition such as cancer and chronic infections. People who are sensitive to cold will sometimes develop hives, asthma, nasal stuffiness, and swollen tissues under the skin.

Cholinergic urticarial is a condition resulting in itchy hives with redness around them. It is usually triggered by sensitivity to heat and any activity that causes sweating.

How do doctors diagnose this condition?

Studies are underway to find causes of these types of allergies. Some experts think that mistaking proteins is behind the problem. Certain drugs like cosmetics, creams and lotions along with the sunlight could be a link to the physical allergy.

When diagnosing what physical allergy reaction you have it is very important to monitor when the hives appear and what brought them on. The more information you doctor has the better is it to prevent you from going through a serious of test.

If you should break out in hives from being outside in the cold, tell this to your doctor and he can test it by putting an ice cube on your skin for 4 minutes. After removing the ice he can than watch the hives appear. This will tell him how to treat this particular condition

Emotional stress is something we all have at one time or another but not everyone will break out in hives from it. Try to relieve as much stress as possible by avoiding it or maybe learning the technique of Yoga. Tell your doctors what happens when you become emotionally stressed and he can give you medication to help slow the stress down. You can also avoid stressors to keep stress at bay.

How does someone know if they have physical allergies?

You will notice hives come up on your skin with redness around it.

The hives will appear for instance under the armpits or behind the knees after exercising. If you notice hives, be sure to take notice what you were doing at the time they seemed to appear and consult your physician.

Chproheptadine works for the hives from the cold. Hydroxzine is for the hives caused from heat or emotional stress. Avoid the sunlight as much as possible and always use sunscreen when out in it.

How does exercising cause reactions?

Exercising and sweating causes asthma to flare up or hives to appear under the arms, behind the legs, on your face wherever you might me sweating at. Some people only have this reaction when exercising.

Asthma is worsened when you exercise because of the fast breathing that cools and dries the airways. Usually happens more in the cold and dry seasons causing wheezing, difficult to breath, chest feels tight and bringing out hives as well. Stress is the number one factor however that brings on hives.

Do not try self-treatment:

Self-Treatment is not advisable for treating allergies until you know for sure that the symptoms are caused from. Consulting your doctor should be one of the first things to do. He will be able to advise you on the treatment you should be taking. Not all symptoms and conditions are treated alike. Next, learn about food allergies to find relief.

About the Author

Martha Grace Hart was born in New York. She has always lived the high life because of her family's status in society. She was born into an influential family with a businessman of a mother and a doctor of a father.

Growing up, Martha has always had everything she wanted delivered on a silver platter. However, she is limited in terms of physical achievements because of her allergies.

In 1984, Martha became a pediatrician and spent the next 30 years looking after her patients.

Today, Martha spends her time taking care of her family, especially her son, Gerard.